Refuse to Age

The Scientific Approach for Aging Well

HANNAH JONES

Table of Content

1 Slowing Aging Pathways

Introduction

Welcome, intrepid explorers, to the gateway of eternal youth! In this enchanting chapter, we embark on a quest through the mesmerizing realms of slowing down the aging process. Picture a world where the sands of time dare not tread too heavily, and wrinkles are but whispers in the wind.

Join us as we unfurl the secrets concealed within the very fabric of our existence. It's not just about counting the years but rewriting the script of aging itself. Brace yourselves for a revelatory expedition into the key factors and secret pathways that shape the narrative of our aging odyssey.

As we navigate through the corridors of science, prepare to be captivated by the dance of molecules and the symphony of cellular whispers. This is not just a chapter; it's an overture to a grand symposium of longevity. By journey's end, you'll possess the sacred knowledge to defy the relentless march of time.

So, adventurer, fasten your seatbelt, for we are about to embark on a spellbinding journey into the heart of timeless vitality. Let the quest for the Fountain of Youth begin!

AMPK

AMPK: Unlocking Cellular Energy Harmony

Journey into the Molecular Realm

Welcome to the first key destination in our quest to slow down the aging process – AMPK, the molecular maestro orchestrating cellular energy harmony. In this leg of our adventure, we'll unravel the significance of AMPK, a molecular switch that holds the key to unlocking the secrets of vitality and longevity.

The Maestro: AMPK Unveiled

AMPK, or Adenosine Monophosphate-Activated Protein Kinase, is not just a mere molecular switch; it's the virtuoso conductor of the cellular symphony. Picture it as the maestro waving its wand, directing cells in a harmonious dance of energy regulation.

Regulating Cellular Energy: The AMPK Symphony

The magic lies in AMPK's ability to regulate cellular energy. As the conductor of this symphony, AMPK monitors and adjusts the cellular energy status. When energy levels are low, AMPK steps in to restore balance by promoting energy production and inhibiting energy-consuming processes.

Impact on Overall Health: A Cellular Serenade

But why is AMPK's role so crucial in the grand scheme of our health? Activating AMPK doesn't just fine-tune energy production; it also sets in motion a cascade of events that positively impact various aspects of our well-being. From metabolic health to cellular repair, AMPK activation is like a soothing serenade for our cells.

Slowing Down the Aging Process: AMPK as the Timeless Conductor

Here's the pièce de résistance – activating AMPK can be your secret weapon against the ticking clock. By promoting cellular energy efficiency and resilience, AMPK activation has the potential to slow down the aging process, keeping your cells in tune for longer.

So, fellow traveler, let's delve into the intricate world of AMPK, where the molecular dance of energy unfolds, and the symphony of longevity begins. Activate the conductor, and let the timeless melody of cellular vitality commence!

Embarking on a Molecular Journey with AMPK: The Symphony of Longevity

Greetings, fellow voyagers! As we step into the enchanting world of AMPK, envision a molecular realm where the dance of energy unfolds like a mesmerizing ballet. AMPK, our virtuoso conductor, beckons us to witness the symphony of longevity – a timeless melody resonating within the intricate web of our cells.

The Intricate Dance of Energy

Picture AMPK as the choreographer of a grand ballet, where cellular components pirouette in perfect harmony. It's not just about regulating energy; it's a dance that synchronizes the entire cellular orchestra, ensuring every note is played with precision.

Activating the Conductor: A Call to Cellular Harmony

Now, imagine yourself as the conductor's assistant, holding the baton of activation. As you delve into the intricate world of AMPK, you're not just observing; you're participating in the orchestration of vitality. With each activation, you amplify the resonance of cellular harmony, setting the stage for a performance that defies the constraints of time.

The Timeless Melody of Cellular Vitality

As you activate the conductor within, the timeless melody of cellular vitality commences. It's a symphony that echoes through the corridors of your being, influencing not just energy regulation but the very essence of your cellular existence. This melody is the soundtrack of longevity, playing softly in the background as your cells dance through the rhythms of life.

So, fellow travelers, join the cosmic ballet of AMPK activation. Feel the resonance, embrace the harmony, and let the timeless melody of cellular vitality surround you. Together, we embark on a journey where the music of longevity plays on, transcending the boundaries of time and space. Let the symphony unfold, and may your cellular vitality be a timeless masterpiece!

Autophagy

Autophagy: The Body's Marvelous Recycling Symphony

In this segment of our journey into the realms of slowing aging pathways, let's explore the captivating phenomenon of autophagy. Imagine autophagy as the body's own masterful recycling system, tirelessly at work to orchestrate a ballet of renewal and rejuvenation within your cells.

Autophagy Unveiled: Nature's Recycling Maestro

Autophagy, derived from the Greek words "auto" (self) and "phagy" (eating), is a biological masterpiece, akin to a diligent janitor sweeping through the cellular corridors. It's the body's innate ability to identify and dispose of damaged or unnecessary cellular components, ensuring a continuous cycle of regeneration and maintenance.

The Ballet of Cellular Renewal: Autophagy's Dance

Envision your cells engaged in an intricate dance of self-improvement. During autophagy, cellular components deemed past their prime are encapsulated, broken down, and repurposed. This meticulous process not only rids your cells of the old and worn-out but also paves the way for fresh, resilient structures to take their place.

Promoting Cellular Health: Autophagy's Healing Touch

Beyond the poetic dance, autophagy holds profound implications for cellular health. By systematically removing damaged components, it acts as a guardian, shielding your cells from the wear and tear of time. The result? Enhanced cellular resilience and potential longevity, as damaged cells make way for a rejuvenated, more youthful cellular landscape

Extending the Lifespan: Autophagy's Promise

Picture autophagy as a timeless fountain of youth. By actively participating in this natural recycling symphony, you not only promote immediate cellular health but also potentially extend your lifespan. It's as if autophagy whispers to your cells, encouraging them to embrace vitality and endure the passage of time with grace.

Cellular Senescence

Our exploration into the intricate tapestry of slowing aging pathways brings us to the intriguing realm of cellular senescence. Imagine cellular senescence as a twilight state where cells, having served their purpose, find themselves at a crossroads, transitioning from active contributors to silent observers.

Decoding Cellular Senescence: The State of Transition

Cellular senescence is a captivating phenomenon, reminiscent of a wise elder sharing the tales of its journey. It's a state in which cells lose their normal function, entering a period of rest or retirement. Much like a well-earned sabbatical, cellular senescence can be seen as both a conclusion and a new beginning.

Implications Unveiled: The Dance of Cellular Wisdom

As we delve into the implications of managing cellular senescence, envision a dance where aging cells gracefully step aside, making room for the next generation. By understanding and influencing this state of transition, we gain insights into how the aging process can be shaped and molded.

Managing Cellular Senescence: A Key to Healthier Aging

Consider managing cellular senescence as a gentle guide navigating the twilight of cellular function. Just as a wise mentor imparts lessons for future generations, managing senescence becomes a crucial strategy for healthier aging. It involves orchestrating the balance between the old and the new, ensuring a harmonious cellular landscape.

A Symphony of Balance: Shaping the Aging Narrative

In the grand symphony of life, cellular senescence plays a distinctive tune. By exploring its intricacies and implications, we gain the power to influence the aging narrative. Managing cellular senescence becomes an art—a delicate dance that holds the promise of healthier, more vibrant aging.

Embarking on a Cellular Odyssey: Navigating the Twilight of Senescence

Greetings, fellow voyagers! As we set sail into the uncharted waters of cellular senescence, imagine this realm as a twilight sanctuary, where cells share their stories and impart the wisdom acquired through a lifetime of service. Join us on this profound journey of uncovering the tales held within the cellular tapestry and embracing the dance of managing senescence as our guiding compass toward a future of graceful and healthier aging.

Stories of Cellular Legacy: Tales in the Twilight

Picture cellular senescence as a cosmic library, each cell carrying a book filled with its unique narrative. These cells, having played pivotal roles, now enter a state of reflection, sharing their tales of resilience, adaptation, and the intricate dance with time. Uncover the stories woven into the fabric of cellular existence, stories that echo the wisdom gained through the eons.

The Wisdom Within: Lessons Learned in Senescence

As we delve into the twilight realm, acknowledge the profound wisdom held by senescent cells. They whisper secrets of adaptation, resilience, and the intricate art of embracing change. It's a wisdom that transcends the boundaries of time, offering valuable insights into the symphony of life and the delicate balance required for graceful aging.

The Dance of Management: Guiding Cells to Graceful Aging

Embrace the metaphorical dance of managing cellular senescence as we navigate through this twilight sanctuary. Much like a choreographer orchestrating a ballet, we hold the power to guide cells through the graceful movements of aging. By understanding and influencing senescence, we become stewards of a future where the dance is one of resilience, vitality, and sustained well-being.

A Future of Graceful Aging: Following the Cellular Choreography

As we conclude our journey into the twilight realm, envision a future where the dance of managing cellular senescence serves as our guide. Let the wisdom of senescent cells illuminate the path to a time where aging is not a foe but a companion—a dance partner in the symphony of life. May this odyssey be your inspiration for a future of graceful and healthier aging, where each step is a testament to the stories told and the wisdom embraced. Onward, fellow voyagers, to the ageless dance of vitality!

Epigenetics

Epigenetics: Unveiling the Symphony of Genetic Expression

Embark on an exhilarating journey through the captivating landscape of epigenetics, a realm where the language of genes is written not just in the script of DNA but in the intricate annotations of life's experiences. Picture this chapter as an invitation to explore the profound impact of external factors on the orchestration of our genetic symphony, and how the art of understanding and influencing these factors holds the key to crafting a healthier and more vibrant life.

The Essence of Epigenetics: The External Brushstrokes on Genetic Canvas

In the tapestry of our genetic code, epigenetics emerges as the artist's brush, delicately painting layers of influence beyond the basic DNA sequence. External factors, from our environment to lifestyle choices, leave imprints on this canvas, shaping the way our genes express themselves.

The Dance of Gene Expression: A Symphony in Motion

Envision gene expression as a dynamic dance, choreographed by the subtle touches of epigenetic marks. As we explore this dance, we begin to understand how external factors can either amplify or soften the melodies played by our genes. It's a symphony in motion, responding to the intricate cues of our lived experiences.

Understanding the Score: Keys to a Healthier Life

Delve into the profound implications of comprehending and influencing epigenetic factors. It's not merely deciphering the notes of genetic expression but actively participating in crafting the score of a healthier life. By understanding these external influences, we gain the power to fine-tune our genetic symphony toward a more vibrant and resilient future.

Crafting a Healthier and More Vibrant Life: Your Epigenetic Odyssey

Imagine epigenetics as a guide on an odyssey to a healthier and more vibrant life. It's not just a journey through scientific intricacies but a pilgrimage to the core of our existence. By navigating the landscape of epigenetics, we unearth the secrets to harmonizing our genes with the rhythm of a well-lived life.

Embarking on the Epigenetic Odyssey: Crafting a Symphony of Well-being

Greetings, fellow explorers! Join us on a spellbinding journey into the enchanting realm of epigenetics, where every external encounter leaves an indelible mark on the canvas of our genetic existence. Picture this adventure as a quest to unravel the mysteries within, as we navigate the delicate dance of external brushstrokes creating a symphony of genetic expression. As we embark on this odyssey, let the understanding and influence of these factors be our guiding compass, lighting the way to a life that resonates with health, vitality, and vibrancy.

The Enchantment of Epigenetics: A Canvas of Expression

In the realm of epigenetics, imagine each external influence as a brushstroke, shaping the landscape of our genetic symphony. From the air we breathe to the choices we make, every nuance leaves its mark on the intricate canvas of our DNA. This is a place where science meets art, and our genetic code becomes a living masterpiece, responsive to the external melodies of life.

Unraveling the Mysteries: A Quest for Understanding

Our journey delves into the heart of the mysteries within. It's not merely a scientific pursuit but a personal quest to understand the nuances of our own genetic composition. By decoding the subtle language of epigenetics, we gain insights into how external factors influence our genes, and in turn, how we can influence the narrative of our own well-being.

A Compass for Well-being: Navigating the Path to Health and Vitality

May the understanding and influence of these external brushstrokes become our compass on this odyssey. This is not just a trek through scientific landscapes; it's a navigation through the twists and turns of our own health and vitality. With each revelation, we gain the power to actively shape the symphony of our genetic expression, crafting a life that resonates with well-being.

Onward to the Symphony: The Epigenetic Melody of Vitality

With our compass in hand, let's stride onward to the symphony of epigenetic well-being. Every step we take, every choice we make, contributes to the harmonious melody of health and vitality. As we journey through this enchanting realm, may the echoes of our genetic symphony resound with the vibrancy of a life well-lived. Onward, fellow explorers, to the symphony of epigenetic well-being!

Glycation

Glycation: Unraveling the Sweet Intricacies of Aging

Dive into the intricate world of glycation as we continue our exploration of pathways to slow down the aging process. Imagine glycation as a subtle yet profound dance between sugars and proteins, leaving its mark on the canvas of our cells. In this chapter, we unveil the effects of glycation on the aging process and discover the transformative power of reducing glycation for a body that functions with vitality and exhibits a more youthful appearance.

Glycation Unveiled: The Sweet Encounter of Sugars and Proteins

Glycation is not just a chemical reaction; it's a complex interplay between sugars and proteins. Picture it as a gentle caress, where sugars attach themselves to proteins, forming molecules known as advanced glycation end products (AGEs). These AGEs, though natural, can accumulate and contribute to the aging process.

Effects of Glycation: Navigating the Sweet and Sour Symphony of Aging

As we delve into the effects of glycation, envision a symphony playing in your cells. The sugars, like melodic notes, attach to proteins, altering their structure and function. This sweet and sour symphony can lead to the formation of AGEs, contributing to stiffness, wrinkles, and other signs associated with aging.

Reducing Glycation: A Recipe for Youthful Resilience

Now, picture a transformative process where we actively reduce glycation. It's like refining the notes in our cellular symphony, creating a harmonious melody that resonates with resilience. By mitigating the effects of glycation, we set the stage for a body that functions optimally, maintaining a more youthful and vibrant appearance.

A More Youthful Appearance: The Sweet Fruits of Glycation Management

Reducing glycation isn't just a scientific endeavor; it's a journey toward a more youthful appearance. Imagine it as a fountain of youth, where the subtle adjustments in our lifestyle and choices influence the way our cells age. It's a process that goes beyond skin-deep, impacting the very essence of how we feel and look as we traverse the journey of life.

So, fellow explorers, let's delve into the effects of glycation, understanding its symphony in our cells. As we unveil the secrets within, may the quest for reducing glycation become a transformative journey, leading to a body that ages with grace, vitality, and a timeless youthful allure. Onward to the sweet harmony of glycation management!

Embarking on the Glycation Odyssey: A Symphony of Cellular Harmony

Greetings, fellow explorers! Join us on a mesmerizing journey into the effects of glycation, where sugars and proteins engage in a subtle dance within the orchestra of our cells. As we peel back the layers and unravel the secrets concealed within this symphony, envision a transformative quest. May the pursuit of reducing glycation be our guiding star, leading us to a body that ages not with resignation, but with the elegance of grace, the vibrancy of vitality, and a timeless youthful allure. Onward we go, into the sweet harmony of glycation management!

The Glycation Symphony: Understanding the Cellular Notes

Picture our cells as an intricate orchestra, where glycation orchestrates a unique symphony. Sugars and proteins intertwine, creating a melody that echoes through our cellular landscape. As we delve into the effects of glycation, we decipher the notes, understanding how this subtle dance can influence the aging process.

Unveiling the Secrets: A Journey into Cellular Transformation

Our quest takes us deep into the cellular realms, unveiling the secrets of glycation. It's not merely a chemical reaction; it's a narrative written in the language of molecules. As we grasp the intricacies of this symphony, we embark on a transformative journey, armed with the knowledge to shape the way our cells age.

Reducing Glycation: A Symphony of Resilience

Imagine the act of reducing glycation as a conductor refining the notes in our cellular symphony. It's a deliberate effort to create a harmony that resonates with resilience. By managing glycation, we craft a melody that promotes not just external youthfulness but a profound vitality that echoes within the very core of our being.

A Body that Ages with Grace: The Elegance of Glycation Management

The quest for reducing glycation transcends the pursuit of mere aesthetics. It leads us to a vision of a body that ages with grace – a vessel that carries the wisdom of years while radiating the energy of vitality. This is the timeless allure, where the sweet harmony of glycation management becomes the melody of a life well-lived.

IGF-1

GF-1: Harmonizing Growth and the Aging Tapestry

As we venture into the realm of IGF-1, envision this hormone as the masterful architect of growth, shaping the intricate patterns of our biological tapestry. IGF-1, the orchestrator in the grand symphony of life, guides us through the dance of cellular processes, each note resonating with the essence of growth and development. In this chapter, we explore the nuanced role of IGF-1, understanding its profound effects on our body's journey through time, and how cultivating equilibrium in its levels becomes a pivotal factor in influencing the aging process.

IGF-1 Unveiled: The Maestro Behind the Scenes

Behold IGF-1, a silent maestro weaving the threads of our growth narrative. Picture it not just as a conductor but as the unseen hand shaping the very fabric of our physical existence. It's the force that whispers to our cells, signaling for growth and harmonizing the dance of life.

Balancing Growth: A Delicate Choreography with Aging

See IGF-1 levels as nimble dancers, engaged in a delicate waltz with the passage of time. Too exuberant, and the dance might lead to unchecked growth; too restrained, and the rhythm of life might lose its grace. Achieving a harmonious equilibrium in IGF-1 levels becomes an art form, a dance that doesn't defy aging but embraces it with refined poise.

Influence on Aging: IGF-1 as the Timekeeper

In our exploration, we uncover the timeless influence of IGF-1 on the aging process. It's not just a hormone overseeing growth; it's a subtle timekeeper orchestrating the cadence of our later years. Understanding the delicate interplay between IGF-1 and aging provides us with a compass, guiding us toward a narrative of aging that's not measured merely in years but in the symphony of vitality.

Balanced Aging: The Symphony of Equanimity

Consider the pursuit of balanced IGF-1 levels as a quest for symphonic equanimity in the aging composition. It's about attuning our hormonal dance to the natural rhythms of life, creating a melody that resonates with a gracefully balanced existence. By embracing and influencing IGF-1 levels, we aspire not just for longevity but for a rich and nuanced life, where each passing note contributes to a harmonious and vibrant aging tapestry.

Embarking on the IGF-1 Expedition: Crafting the Symphony of Aging Gracefully

Greetings, fellow explorers! Join us as we embark on a captivating journey through the intricate landscapes of IGF-1, where the hormonal maestro choreographs a mesmerizing dance between growth and aging. As we unravel the nuanced role of this conductor, let the quest for balanced IGF-1 levels become not just a scientific pursuit but an artistic endeavor—a canvas upon which we craft a life that ages with the elegance of a well-conducted symphony. Onward we go, into the exploration of IGF-1 and the artistry of balanced aging!

IGF-1: The Maestro in the Dance of Time

Imagine IGF-1 as the unseen maestro directing the grand ballet of growth and aging. It orchestrates a dance that unfolds within the very fabric of our existence. Each note, each movement, resonates with the passage of time, creating a symphony that encapsulates the essence of life's evolving rhythms.

Traversing Intricate Landscapes: Unveiling IGF-1's Canvas

As we traverse the intricate landscapes, envision IGF-1 as the painter of our aging canvas. Its brushstrokes delicately influence the pace of growth, leaving imprints that echo through the years. The exploration of IGF-1 becomes a journey into the artistry of existence, where every molecular nuance contributes to the creation of a masterpiece.

The Artistic Endeavor: Balancing the IGF-1 Palette

Consider the quest for balanced IGF-1 levels as our artistic endeavor. It's akin to finding the perfect blend of colors on a palette—a delicate balance that shapes the portrait of aging. By understanding and influencing IGF-1, we become artists crafting not just longevity but a life that unfolds with the finesse of a well-conducted symphony.

Crafting a Life with Elegance: Aging as a Masterpiece

May the pursuit of balanced IGF-1 levels be our artistic expression in the grand gallery of life. It's more than a scientific exploration; it's an opportunity to craft a life that ages with elegance, resilience, and timeless allure. In the exploration of IGF-1, we discover the artistry of balanced aging—a masterpiece in the making.

Inflammation

Inflammation: Navigating the Fires Within

Our expedition into the pathways of slowing aging now leads us to the fiery realm of inflammation. Picture inflammation not just as a response but as a dynamic force influencing the aging process. In this chapter, we delve into the profound impact of chronic inflammation, understanding its role as a catalyst for aging. Join us as we explore effective strategies to manage inflammation, unlocking the gateway to overall health and well-being.

Inflammation Explored: The Dynamic Dance of Immune Response

Envision inflammation as a dynamic dance within the body, an intricate response orchestrated by the immune system. It's not merely a reaction but a conversation—a dialogue between our cells and the environment. Chronic inflammation, however, transforms this dance into a relentless force, becoming a significant player in the aging narrative.

Chronic Inflammation: The Unwanted Guest in the Aging Symphony

As we navigate the impact of chronic inflammation, recognize it as the unwanted guest that overstays its welcome. Prolonged inflammation becomes a disruptor, contributing to a host of age-related issues, from joint discomfort to increased vulnerability to diseases. Understanding its role is the first step in reclaiming control over the aging symphony.

Managing the Flames: Strategies for Inflammation Control

Picture inflammation management as wielding a skilled hand over the flames. By exploring ways to mitigate chronic inflammation, we regain mastery over the aging process. Lifestyle adjustments, dietary choices, and mindful practices emerge as tools to quell the flames, promoting a harmonious balance within the body.

Promoting Well-being: The Anti-Inflammatory Odyssey

Consider the quest for inflammation management as an odyssey towards well-being. It's not a battle against the body but a journey to restore equilibrium. By adopting practices that soothe the inflammatory fires, we pave the way for overall health—physically, mentally, and emotionally.

So, fellow explorers, let's journey into the realm of inflammation, where the fires within shape the narrative of aging. As we uncover the impact of chronic inflammation, may the quest for its management become our guiding light—a path towards a life where well-being prevails, and the symphony of aging plays with the grace of harmony.

Onward to the exploration of inflammation and the art of aging gracefully!

Embarking on the Inflammatory Expedition: Crafting the Symphony of Graceful Aging

Greetings, fellow explorers! Join us as we embark on a transformative journey into the intricate realm of inflammation, where the fires within weave the narrative of aging. In this chapter, let us unravel the impact of chronic inflammation, acknowledging it as a pivotal force that shapes the story of our aging journey. May the quest for inflammation management be our guiding light—a pathway leading us toward a life where well-being prevails, and the symphony of aging unfolds with the elegance of harmony. Onward we go, into the exploration of inflammation and the art of aging gracefully!

Inflammation's Realm: The Fires Shaping Aging's Tale

Imagine inflammation as a realm where fires dance within, influencing the very essence of aging. It's a dynamic landscape, with each flame representing the body's response to the intricacies of life. Chronic inflammation, however, transforms this landscape into a story of imbalance, impacting the aging process in profound ways.

Chronic Inflammation Unveiled: A Disruptive Force in the Aging Symphony

As we venture deeper, chronic inflammation emerges as a disruptive force—a relentless guest that alters the harmony of the aging symphony. Its prolonged presence becomes a narrative thread, weaving discomfort and vulnerability into the tapestry of our later years. Uncovering its impact is the first step toward reclaiming control over the aging narrative.

Guiding Light of Management: Illuminating the Path to Well-being

Picture inflammation management as a guiding light in the dark expanse of chronic inflammation. It's not a battle against the body but a journey to restore equilibrium. By exploring strategies to quell the inflammatory flames—be it through lifestyle adjustments or mindful practices—we set forth on a path where well-being becomes the prevailing theme.

The Anti-Inflammatory Odyssey: Paving the Way to Harmony

Consider the quest for inflammation management as an odyssey toward harmony—a journey where each step is a note in the symphony of well-being. It's an artful exploration, where the body, mind, and spirit align in a dance that echoes with grace. The flames are not extinguished but tempered, creating a canvas where the art of aging gracefully takes center stage.

Oxidation

Oxidation: Navigating the Balance of Life's Fire

Embark with us on a journey into the intricate realm of Oxidation, a chapter where the concept of oxidative stress reveals its impact on the aging process. Picture oxidation not merely as a chemical reaction but as the dance of life's fire within our cells. In this exploration, we unravel the profound effects of oxidative stress and discover the art of managing it—an endeavor that holds the key to cultivating a more resilient and youthful body.

Oxidative Stress Unveiled: Life's Dance with Fire

Envision oxidative stress as the dance of fire within our cellular landscape—an inherent part of life's intricate balance. The oxygen that sustains us can also, paradoxically, contribute to cellular damage. As we delve into oxidative stress, we comprehend its role in the aging narrative, a story where unchecked flames can accelerate the aging process.

Impact on Aging: The Unseen Threads of Oxidative Influence

Navigate through the unseen threads woven by oxidative stress, impacting the aging journey in subtle ways. From cellular damage to the manifestation of age-related conditions, oxidative stress becomes a silent contributor to the chapters of our lives. Understanding its influence is akin to deciphering the language of our cells, offering insights into the aging symphony.

Managing Oxidative Stress: A Journey to Resilience

Imagine managing oxidative stress as a journey to build resilience—a quest not to extinguish the flames of life but to balance them. Through lifestyle choices, dietary decisions, and mindful practices, we navigate the path toward a more harmonious oxidative dance. It's an artful endeavor, crafting a body that withstands the tests of time with vitality and youthfulness.

Contribution to Youthful Vigor: The Symphony of Balanced Oxidation

Consider the quest to manage oxidative stress as the conductor's baton shaping a symphony of balanced oxidation. It's not about eliminating life's fire but orchestrating it in a way that preserves youthful vigor. The journey holds the promise of a body resilient to the effects of time, aging with a grace that echoes through the years.

So, fellow explorers, let's delve into the realm of Oxidation, where the dance of life's fire shapes the narrative of aging. As we explore the impact of oxidative stress, may the quest for its management become an artful journey—a path toward a more resilient and youthful body. Onward to the exploration of Oxidation and the symphony of aging with resilience and grace!

Telomeres

Telomeres: Architects of Cellular Destiny and Aging Chronicles

In the intricate tapestry of cellular life, telomeres emerge as central architects, orchestrating the fate of cells and weaving the narrative of aging. These protective caps, composed of nucleotide repeats, serve as guardians at the ends of chromosomes, ensuring a delicate balance between responding to stress, fostering growth, and managing the repercussions of cellular history.

To avoid the activation of DNA repair pathways, telomeres must extend a protective shield, with at least a few hundred nucleotides forming a cap at each chromosome end. The repair mechanisms for critically short or "uncapped" telomeres are limited in most somatic cells. When an excess of these vulnerable telomeres accumulates, the cellular fate takes a decisive turn, leading to apoptosis or cellular senescence—a phenomenon triggered by the limitations in repairing these delicate ends.

The chance of encountering cellular senescence amplifies as the average telomere length diminishes. In the realm of germline cells, where telomerase expression is abundant, the average telomere length is set and vigilantly maintained. However, in the heterogeneous landscape of somatic cells, telomere length typically declines with age. This dual role—acting as a barrier to tumor growth while contributing to the loss of cells with age—paints telomeres as both defenders and contributors to the aging saga.

The attrition of (stem) cells due to telomere shortening introduces a powerful selection force favoring abnormal and malignant cells. This process is further fueled by genome instability and aneuploidy triggered by dysfunctional telomeres. The indispensable role of telomeres in orchestrating cell turnover and aging is poignantly underscored by patients with 50% of normal telomerase levels, resulting from mutations in telomerase genes.

In this altered scenario, short telomeres become implicated in various disorders, including dyskeratosis congenita, aplastic anemia, pulmonary fibrosis, and cancer. The complex interplay of telomeres and telomerase in human aging and aging-associated diseases invites a profound review of their roles. As we unravel the tales written in the telomeres, we gain insights into the intricate dance between cellular destiny and the aging chronicles, where telomeres emerge as both architects and narrators of the story etched in the cellular landscape.

22. Optimal Anti-Aging Lifestyle

Diet

Embark with us on a transformative journey into the realm of optimal anti-aging lifestyle, where the spotlight shines on the profound impact of nutrition on the aging process. In this chapter, we unravel the secrets of diets that stand the test of time, exploring the culinary traditions of centenarians and delving into the Mediterranean and Okinawan diets. Let's also unveil the phenomenon of the Red, White, and Blue Zone, while discovering the myriad benefits of embracing a plant-based diet—a key to unlocking the door to a longer, healthier life.

Nutrient-Rich Odyssey: Diets of Centenarians

Venture into the dietary realms of those who defy the hands of time—centenarians. Their diets, often rich in specific nutrients and balanced proportions, serve as a blueprint for aging with vitality. By understanding their culinary choices, we glean insights into the power of nutrition in promoting longevity and well-being.

Mediterranean Magic: Savoring Life's Elixir

Explore the enchanting Mediterranean diet, renowned for its heart-healthy components and longevity-promoting properties. Immerse yourself in the world of olive oil, fresh vegetables, whole grains, and lean proteins, and discover how this culinary tradition weaves a tapestry of health, flavor, and timeless well-being.

Okinawan Wisdom: Aging with Grace and Vitality

Journey to the shores of Okinawa, where longevity is not just a concept but a way of life. Uncover the secrets of the Okinawan diet, where nutrient-dense foods like sweet potatoes, seaweed, and tofu take center stage. The wisdom embedded in their dietary choices offers a glimpse into aging with grace and vitality.

Red, White, and Blue Zone: A Tapestry of Health

Dive into the phenomenon of the Red, White, and Blue Zone—a captivating exploration of regions where the elixir of life seems to flow abundantly. Through dietary patterns and lifestyle choices, these zones provide valuable lessons on how food can become a fountain of youth, contributing to the longevity and well-being of their inhabitants.

Plant-Powered Resilience: A Green Path to Longevity

Delve into the benefits of embracing a plant-based diet, where the vibrancy of fruits, vegetables, legumes, and nuts takes center stage. Unlock the potential of plant-powered resilience, discovering how these nutrient-rich foods contribute not only to physical health but also to a longer, more vibrant life.

As we navigate the dietary landscape of optimal anti-aging lifestyles, may this exploration be a source of inspiration. By incorporating the wisdom gleaned from centenarians, embracing the Mediterranean and

Okinawan traditions, decoding the secrets of the Red, White, and Blue Zone, and reveling in the nourishment of plant-based delights, we pave the way to a future where aging is synonymous with timeless well-being. Onward to the exploration of optimal nutrition, where the journey to a longer, healthier life begins with the choices we make on our plates!

Beverages

In this chapter of the optimal anti-aging lifestyle, let's take a refreshing detour into the world of beverages—a liquid symphony that holds the potential to orchestrate anti-aging effects. Here, we dive into the science behind certain drinks, unlocking their secrets and understanding how they contribute to the elixir of overall well-being.

Hydration Harmony: The Foundation of Wellness

Embark on the journey of hydration, the cornerstone of well-being. Discover how adequate water intake not only quenches our thirst but also plays a vital role in maintaining optimal bodily functions. Hydration, often overlooked, is a fundamental elixir that supports the body's resilience against the sands of time.

Tea Time Elegance: Antioxidant-rich Infusions

Indulge in the elegance of tea—a timeless beverage celebrated for more than just its taste. Uncover the antioxidant-rich profile of various teas, from green to black, and delve into the potential benefits they offer. As we sip these infusions, we tap into the power of antioxidants, guarding our cells against oxidative stress and contributing to the anti-aging tapestry.

Coffee Chronicles: Beyond the Morning Pick-Me-Up

Navigate the coffee chronicles, where the beloved morning pick-me-up transcends its role. Explore the scientific nuances of coffee, understanding its potential anti-aging effects. From antioxidant properties to cognitive benefits, coffee emerges as a beverage not just for stimulation but as a companion in the journey to timeless wellness.

Nectar of Nature: Juices and Beyond

Venture into the realm of natural juices—a nectar bestowed upon us by nature. Unveil the potential benefits of fruit and vegetable juices, rich in vitamins, minerals, and phytonutrients. These vibrant elixirs contribute not only to hydration but also to a nutrient-packed arsenal supporting our bodies in the quest for anti-aging resilience.

Beyond the Glass: The Science of Beverage Wellness

As we explore the role of beverages in the optimal anti-aging lifestyle, it's essential to understand the science that underpins their effects. From maintaining hydration harmony to unlocking the antioxidant prowess of teas and coffees, and savoring the nectar of nature through juices, each sip becomes a step toward timeless wellness.

May this journey into the realm of beverages be a reminder that our choices in what we drink can be a powerful elixir, influencing not only our physical well-being but also contributing to the symphony of anti-aging effects. Onward to the exploration of the science and artistry behind beverages, where each sip becomes a celebration of timeless wellness!

Lifestyle

In the pursuit of optimal aging, the chapter on lifestyle unfolds as a garden of choices, where each decision becomes a seed planted for timeless vitality. Let's immerse ourselves in the essential lifestyle factors that pave the way for optimal well-being, embracing the importance of regular exercise, maintaining a healthy weight, prioritizing quality sleep, effective stress management, and nurturing social ties.

1. Exercise: Nurturing the Body and Mind

Embark on the journey of regular exercise—a cornerstone of the optimal anti-aging lifestyle. Whether it's a brisk walk, a joyful dance, or a purposeful workout, exercise brings a cascade of benefits. It enhances cardiovascular health, strengthens muscles and bones, and uplifts mood through the release of endorphins. The dance between body and mind during exercise is a symphony that contributes to the overall vibrancy of life.

2. Weight Control: Balancing the Scales of Well-being

Maintaining a healthy weight becomes a pivotal brushstroke in the canvas of optimal aging. Beyond aesthetics, weight control is a key contributor to preventing chronic conditions associated with aging, such as heart disease and diabetes. It's an investment in the body's resilience, ensuring that the scales tip in favor of long-term health.

3. Sleep: The Restorative Elixir of Night

Prioritize quality sleep as the restorative elixir that replenishes the body and mind. Adequate and restful sleep is essential for cellular repair, cognitive function, and emotional well-being. In the realm of optimal aging, each night's sleep becomes a canvas upon which the body paints the colors of rejuvenation.

4. Stress Management: Crafting Serenity in a Busy World

Navigate the art of stress management—a skill that becomes increasingly valuable in the tapestry of optimal aging. Whether through mindfulness practices, meditation, or other relaxation techniques, effective stress management contributes to a more peaceful and centered existence. It's a shield against the wear and tear of daily challenges, fostering emotional resilience.

5. Social Ties: Weaving the Fabric of Fulfillment

Nurture social ties as threads that weave the fabric of a fulfilling and vibrant life. Meaningful connections with friends, family, and community contribute to emotional well-being and provide a support system during life's ups and downs. Social ties, often underestimated, are essential elements in the symphony of optimal aging.

As we navigate the landscape of lifestyle factors for optimal anti-aging, may these choices become intentional steps toward a more fulfilling and vibrant life. Whether it's the rhythm of exercise, the balance of weight control, the restorative nature of sleep, the art of stress management, or the warmth of social ties, each element plays a crucial role in cultivating the seeds of timeless vitality. Onward to the exploration of an optimal lifestyle, where each choice becomes a brushstroke in the masterpiece of aging with grace and vibrancy!

III. Function Preservation

Bones

Nurturing Resilience in Your Bones

In the journey of aging, the chapter on preserving bone health emerges as a crucial guide, offering insights into effective strategies for maintaining the strength and resilience of your skeletal structure. Let's take a deep dive into the world of bone health, unraveling the interplay of nutrition, exercise, and lifestyle habits that become the cornerstone of preserving function and ensuring your bones stand the test of time.

Nutrition for Bone Resilience: Building from Within

Embark on a nutritional journey that lays the foundation for resilient bones. Calcium, vitamin D, and other essential nutrients are the building blocks that fortify your skeletal structure. From dairy products to leafy greens, a well-balanced diet becomes the nourishment that strengthens your bones from within.

Exercise: The Symphony of Skeletal Strength

Participate in the symphony of skeletal strength through targeted exercises. Weight-bearing activities, resistance training, and flexibility exercises become the notes that resonate within your bones, promoting bone density and preventing age-related bone loss.

The dance between muscles and bones becomes a harmonious partnership, enhancing overall skeletal well-being.

Lifestyle Habits: A Blueprint for Bone Wellness

Craft a blueprint for bone wellness through mindful lifestyle habits. Avoiding excessive alcohol consumption and refraining from smoking contribute to bone health. These habits, when integrated into your daily life, act as guardians, protecting your bones from the detrimental effects of harmful substances.

Strategies for Aging Gracefully: Preserving Your Bones for a Lifetime

As you age, adopting strategies for preserving your bones becomes an investment in a lifetime of mobility and vitality. Regular weight-bearing exercises, coupled with a diet rich in bone-supporting nutrients, create a powerful synergy. Avoiding sedentary habits and embracing an active lifestyle further fortify your skeletal foundation.

Embrace Bone Density Screening: Knowledge as a Shield

In the pursuit of preserving bone function, consider embracing bone density screening as a shield against potential challenges. Early detection of bone density issues allows for proactive measures, ensuring timely interventions to maintain and enhance bone health.

As you delve into the realm of preserving your bones, may this exploration be a guide to nurturing resilience and strength. From the nutritional choices that build your bones from within to the symphony of exercises that resonate through your skeletal structure, each step becomes a dance toward aging with grace. Onward to the preservation of function, where your bones become the pillars supporting a life of vitality and well-being!

Bowel and Bladder Function

Nurturing Bowel and Bladder Wellness for Lifelong Vitality

In the mosaic of preserving function, the spotlight turns towards the often overlooked yet essential realms of bowel and bladder health. Let's embark on a journey into the intricacies of maintaining these vital functions, unraveling the factors that influence digestive health, and discovering practices to support optimal functioning for a life of enduring vitality.

Understanding Digestive Dynamics: The Foundation of Wellness

To preserve the function of bowel and bladder, we first delve into the complex dance of digestive dynamics. A healthy digestive system is not only instrumental in nutrient absorption but also plays a crucial role in maintaining overall well-being. From the intricate web of the gut microbiome to the mechanics of peristalsis, understanding these processes becomes the key to preserving lifelong function.

Factors Influencing Digestive Health: Unveiling the Tapestry

Explore the factors that influence digestive health, ranging from dietary choices to hydration, stress levels, and physical activity. Each element woven into the tapestry of digestive wellness contributes to the overall harmony of bowel and bladder function. Recognizing and addressing these factors lay the groundwork for preserving optimal function as we age.

Practices for Optimal Functioning: Nurturing Your Internal Ecosystem

Discover practices that nurture your internal ecosystem, promoting bowel and bladder health throughout life. Dietary considerations, such as fiber-rich foods and proper hydration, become allies in maintaining regularity and preventing digestive discomfort. Mindful eating practices and stress management techniques contribute to a balanced digestive system, fostering a resilient foundation for long-term wellness.

The Mind-Body Connection: Stress, Digestion, and Well-being

Acknowledge the intricate relationship between stress and digestive health. Chronic stress can impact bowel and bladder function, highlighting the importance of stress management techniques. Mindfulness practices, relaxation exercises, and fostering a supportive mental environment become integral components in the preservation of optimal function.

Empowering Your Future Self: A Lifelong Commitment to Digestive Health

As we explore the nuances of preserving bowel and bladder function, let this journey be a commitment to empowering your future self. The choices made today, from mindful eating to stress management, serve as investments in a life of enduring vitality. By understanding the intricacies of digestive dynamics and implementing practices for optimal functioning, we lay the foundation for a future where the symphony of bodily functions plays on with grace and resilience.

Onward to the exploration of preserving function, where the nurturing of bowel and bladder wellness becomes a testament to the artistry of aging with enduring vitality!

Circulation

Nurturing the Lifeblood - Your Circulation

In the journey of aging, the chapter on preserving function unfolds as a testament to the intricate dance of bodily systems. Within this tapestry, the spotlight shines on the paramount importance of preserving circulation—a lifeline that fuels every cell and ensures the vitality of the body. Let's delve into the significance of maintaining good circulation for overall health and explore the lifestyle choices and habits that become the architects of a robust circulatory system.

The Symphony of Circulation: A Vital Rhythm for Well-being

Circulation, often likened to the symphony of life, orchestrates the flow of nutrients, oxygen, and life force to every nook and cranny of the body. It's a rhythm that, when uninterrupted, sustains the vitality of organs, tissues, and cells. Preserving this symphony becomes a key melody in the composition of a healthy and vibrant existence.

Lifestyle Choices: The Brushstrokes of Circulatory Health

Embrace lifestyle choices that serve as brushstrokes, painting a portrait of circulatory well-being. Regular physical activity emerges as a hero, promoting blood flow, strengthening the heart, and enhancing the flexibility of blood vessels. Whether through aerobic exercises, brisk walks, or yoga, each movement contributes to the dance of circulation.

Nutrition: Fueling the Circulatory Engine

Explore the role of nutrition as the fuel for the circulatory engine. Diets rich in fruits, vegetables, whole grains, and lean proteins provide the nutrients necessary for maintaining optimal blood viscosity and supporting arterial health. Adequate hydration also ensures the fluidity of blood, allowing it to traverse the intricate pathways of the circulatory system with ease.

Avoiding Tobacco and Limiting Alcohol: Clearing the Pathways

Consider the impact of lifestyle habits on circulatory health. Tobacco, with its detrimental effects on blood vessels, is a roadblock to optimal circulation. Similarly, excessive alcohol consumption can strain the circulatory system. Clearing these pathways by avoiding tobacco and moderating alcohol intake becomes a conscious choice in preserving circulation.

Regular Health Check-ups: The Compass for Circulatory Wellness

Engage in regular health check-ups as a compass guiding circulatory wellness. Monitoring blood pressure, cholesterol levels, and other circulatory markers allows for early detection and intervention, preventing potential issues and ensuring the ongoing symphony of circulation.

Stress Management: Unwinding the Tension in Circulation

Recognize the impact of stress on circulation and embrace stress management techniques as a means of unwinding the tension. Practices such as deep breathing, meditation, or engaging in activities that bring joy contribute to a relaxed circulatory state, fostering overall well-being.

As we navigate the realm of preserving circulation, may these insights be the compass guiding us toward habits and choices that nurture the lifeblood of the body. Whether through movement, nutrition, avoiding harmful substances, regular check-ups, or stress management, each choice becomes a brushstroke in the masterpiece of circulatory well-being. Onward to the exploration of a life where circulation thrives, and the symphony of vitality plays on!

Hair

Nourishing the Crown - A Guide to Ageless Hair

In the intricate tapestry of aging gracefully, the chapter on preserving function extends its embrace to a captivating aspect—preserving the crown of one's glory, the hair. Let's delve into the secrets that unveil the path to maintaining healthy and vibrant locks as the years gracefully unfold. Explore the pivotal roles of nutrition, proper care, and lifestyle choices in the art of preserving your hair.

Nourishment from Within: The Role of Nutrition

Embark on a journey where the sustenance of healthy hair begins from within. Nutrition plays a pivotal role in preserving the vitality of your locks. Explore a diet rich in essential vitamins, minerals, and proteins that act as the building blocks for strong and lustrous hair. From leafy greens to omega-3 fatty acids, each nutrient becomes a brushstroke in the masterpiece of ageless hair.

Proper Care: Tending to the Tresses with Precision

Unlock the secrets of proper care—an art that involves understanding your hair type and tailoring care routines accordingly. From choosing the right shampoo and conditioner to embracing the beauty of occasional hair masks, the ritual of care becomes a tribute to the health and resilience of your locks. Proper care extends beyond aesthetics; it becomes a language of love spoken to your hair.

Lifestyle Choices: Weaving the Fabric of Vibrant Hair

In the tapestry of lifestyle choices, every decision becomes a thread that weaves the fabric of vibrant hair. Manage stress levels, as chronic stress can impact hair health. Embrace a physically active lifestyle that promotes circulation, ensuring that the nutrients reach the hair follicles. Hydration becomes a source of nourishment, keeping your locks resilient and glowing.

As you navigate the realm of preserving your hair, may this exploration be a guide to cultivating ageless locks. The symphony of nutrition, proper care, and lifestyle choices becomes a melody that resonates with the vibrancy of your hair. Onward to the preservation of this cherished crown, where the secrets to ageless hair are unveiled—one strand at a time.

Hearing

*Harmonizing Your Auditory Symphony***

In the symphony of preserving function, let's focus our attention on a key instrument—your hearing. Discover the delicate factors that influence hearing health and explore strategies to ensure the longevity of your auditory function throughout the journey of aging.

Preserving Your Hearing: The Soundtrack of a Well-lived Life

Hearing, often taken for granted, is a symphony that enriches our experiences and connects us to the world. To preserve this vital sense, it's essential to understand the factors that impact hearing health.

Factors Influencing Hearing Health: Unraveling the Melody of Preservation

Explore the intricate melody of factors that can influence hearing health. From exposure to loud noises and environmental factors to genetic predispositions, understanding the nuances of these elements is the first step in preserving your auditory well-being.

Strategies for Optimal Auditory Function: A Symphony of Preservation

Dive into a symphony of strategies designed to maintain optimal auditory function as you age.

- **Protective Measures:** Embrace protective measures such as earplugs or noise-canceling headphones in environments with loud noises. These simple steps can shield your ears from potential damage.

- *Regular Hearing Check-ups:* Schedule regular check-ups with an audiologist to monitor your hearing health. Early detection of issues allows for timely interventions, preventing further deterioration.

- *Healthy Lifestyle Choices:* Adopt a lifestyle that supports overall well-being, as it inevitably contributes to hearing health. A balanced diet, regular exercise, and avoiding excessive exposure to loud sounds all play a part in the symphony of auditory preservation.

- *Mindful Listening:* Cultivate the art of mindful listening. Being aware of your environment and making conscious choices to reduce exposure to loud noises can significantly contribute to the preservation of your hearing.

The Art of Aging with Vibrant Hearing: Preserving Your Auditory Legacy

As you navigate the chapters of life, envision preserving your hearing as an art—an art that contributes to the vibrancy of your overall well-being. By unraveling the factors that influence hearing health and embracing strategies for preservation, you craft a symphony that resonates with the richness of a well-lived life.

May the exploration of strategies for preserving your hearing become a harmonious journey—one that safeguards your auditory legacy and allows you to savor the intricate melodies of life well into the golden years. Onward to the preservation of your auditory function, where each note becomes a testament to aging with grace and vibrancy!

Hormones

*Nurturing the Harmony of Hormonal Well-being***

In the pursuit of preserving function for old age, the chapter on "Preserving Your Hormones" unfolds as a delicate symphony, where the orchestrators of our physiological harmony take center stage. Let's delve into the understanding of hormones in the aging process and explore ways to support hormonal balance for overall well-being—a key to preserving function and vitality in the golden years.

Unlocking the Symphony: The Role of Hormones in Aging

Hormones, the messengers of our biological orchestra, play a pivotal role in shaping the narrative of aging. From regulating metabolism and energy levels to influencing mood and maintaining reproductive health, hormones are the conductors that guide the intricate dance of our physiological functions. Understanding their role becomes a crucial step in preserving function as the years unfold.

The Elegance of Balance: Supporting Hormonal Harmony

Preserving hormonal function is not about halting the natural aging process but about fostering a delicate balance. Explore the ways to support hormonal harmony, acknowledging that fluctuations are a part of the journey. From lifestyle choices to dietary considerations, each decision becomes a note in the symphony, contributing to the overall well-being and preserving the function of these vital messengers.

Nourishment for Hormonal Resilience: Dietary Considerations

Dive into the realm of dietary considerations that nourish hormonal resilience. Certain nutrients and foods can positively impact hormone production and balance. From omega-3 fatty acids for brain health to phytoestrogens for hormonal support, the choices we make on our plates become a form of self-care, nurturing the hormonal symphony for long-term well-being.

Lifestyle Harmony: Exercise, Sleep, and Stress Management

Beyond nutrition, lifestyle factors play a significant role in supporting hormonal balance. Regular exercise, quality sleep, and effective stress management contribute to the harmonious dance of hormones. Exercise, in particular, stimulates the release of endorphins and supports metabolic health, while restful sleep becomes a crucial period of rejuvenation. Stress management techniques, such as mindfulness and relaxation practices, offer a sanctuary for hormonal equilibrium.

The Wisdom of Aging: Embracing Change with Grace

Preserving function for old age is not about resisting change but embracing it with grace and intention. Recognizing that hormonal fluctuations are a natural part of the aging process allows for a more mindful and empowered approach. By understanding the role of hormones and adopting lifestyle and dietary practices that support their balance, we nurture the seeds of vitality, contributing to a life that ages with resilience and well-being.

So, as we explore the delicate symphony of "Preserving Your Hormones," let it be a reminder that preserving function for old age is a nuanced dance— one where understanding, nourishment, and lifestyle choices become the steps toward a harmonious and vibrant journey through the golden years. Onward to the exploration of hormonal well-being, where each note is a gesture of care towards the symphony of aging with grace!

Immune System

In the realm of preserving function, a pivotal chapter unfolds—dedicated to nurturing the guardian within, our immune system. As we delve into the intricacies of this complex defense mechanism, we uncover the keys to bolstering its function. This exploration is not just about safeguarding against illness but also about laying the foundation for longevity and a thriving existence in old age.

Preserving Your Immune System: The Guardian of Longevity

The immune system stands as the vigilant guardian, a complex network of cells, tissues, and organs working harmoniously to protect the body against invaders. To preserve its function is to invest in a shield that not only defends against illness but also contributes to the longevity puzzle.

Understanding the Immune Symphony: A Dance of Defense

Embark on a journey into the symphony of the immune system, where a dance of defense unfolds. Understanding the intricacies of immune responses, from the recognition of pathogens to the deployment of antibodies, empowers us to play an active role in preserving this intricate guardian.

Bolstering Immune Function: Keys to Longevity

Discover the keys to bolstering immune function, paving the way for a life that thrives with vitality even in old age. Nutrition, regular exercise, proper sleep, and stress management emerge as crucial elements in this endeavor. Each choice made in these realms becomes a note in the melody of immune resilience.

Nutritional Nourishment: Fuel for the Guardian

Explore the role of nutrition as fuel for the immune guardian. Nutrient-rich foods, abundant in vitamins and minerals, become the building blocks for a robust immune response. From colorful fruits and vegetables to lean proteins, the choices we make in our diet become a source of strength for the guardian within.

Exercise: Mobilizing the Defense Troops

Regular exercise emerges as a powerful conductor, mobilizing the defense troops within the immune system. Physical activity not only enhances circulation but also contributes to the optimal functioning of immune cells. The rhythmic dance of exercise becomes a choreography that keeps the immune symphony in harmony.

Quality Sleep: The Restoration of Guardian Vigilance

Prioritize quality sleep as the restoration of guardian vigilance. Adequate and restful sleep is a cornerstone in immune function, allowing the body to repair, regenerate, and prepare for the challenges that lie ahead. In the silent hours of the night, the immune system rejuvenates, ensuring its readiness for the days to come.

Stress Management: A Soothing Melody for the Guardian

Navigate the art of stress management as a soothing melody for the immune guardian. Chronic stress can undermine immune function, making stress-reducing practices, such as mindfulness and relaxation techniques, essential for preserving the integrity of the guardian within.

As we journey through the intricacies of preserving function, may the exploration of immune preservation become a conscious effort toward longevity. The choices we make in nourishing our bodies, engaging in regular exercise, prioritizing quality sleep, and managing stress contribute not only to a robust immune system but also to a life that blossoms with vitality in old age. Onward to the preservation of our immune guardian, paving the way for a journey that transcends time with resilience and well-being!

Joints

*A Symphony of Joint Health***

In the chapter dedicated to preserving function, let's journey into the intricate world of joint health—a vital component in the orchestration of a life that ages with grace and mobility. Here, we unravel effective strategies for maintaining flexibility and reducing the risk of age-related joint issues, ensuring that the symphony of movement continues to play harmoniously into old age.

Preserving Your Joints: A Dance of Resilience

Delve into the dance of joint health, where the intricate movements of the body find their rhythm. Joints, the connectors of bones, are essential for mobility and flexibility. As we age, the wear and tear on joints can become more pronounced, making the preservation of joint function a key consideration for a life that remains vibrant and active.

Strategies for Maintaining Flexibility: The Fluidity of Movement

Explore effective strategies for maintaining flexibility—a cornerstone of joint health. Stretching exercises, yoga, and gentle movements become the tools in the hands of those seeking to nurture the fluidity of joint motion. These practices not only enhance flexibility but also contribute to the overall well-being of the musculoskeletal system.

Reducing the Risk of Age-Related Joint Issues: A Preventive Symphony

Uncover the preventive symphony that reduces the risk of age-related joint issues. From maintaining a healthy weight to incorporating joint-friendly exercises, the choices we make play a significant role in preserving the integrity of our joints. By embracing a proactive approach to joint health, we lay the foundation for a future where movement remains a source of joy and freedom.

Holistic Approaches to Joint Care: Beyond Exercise

Recognize that preserving joint function extends beyond exercise alone. Adequate nutrition, hydration, and joint-friendly habits contribute to the holistic well-being of our joints. Nutrients like omega-3 fatty acids and collagen, coupled with proper hydration, become allies in the quest for joint resilience, ensuring that the joints are nourished from within.

Embracing Longevity Through Joint Preservation

As we delve into the strategies for preserving joint function, it becomes clear that joint health is not just about managing issues as they arise but proactively nurturing the resilience of our joints. Each mindful choice becomes a step toward embracing longevity, allowing us to savor the movements of life well into old age.

In the symphony of preserving function, may the dance of joint health be a melody that resonates through the years. By incorporating strategies for maintaining flexibility, reducing the risk of age-related joint issues, and embracing holistic approaches to joint care, we craft a future where each step is a testament to the preservation of function and the celebration of a life in motion. Onward to the exploration of joint health, where the symphony of movement unfolds with grace and resilience!

Mind

Nurturing the Mind for Timeless Brilliance*

In the tapestry of optimal aging, the chapter on preserving function unfolds as a sanctuary for the mind—a realm where cognitive health takes center stage. Join us on a transformative journey into the strategies and practices that preserve and enhance your mental faculties, creating a foundation for timeless brilliance as you age.

Preserving Your Mind: The Gateway to Cognitive Vitality

Embark on a voyage into the intricate landscapes of cognitive health, recognizing the mind as the gateway to timeless brilliance. Preserving your mind involves a holistic approach that nurtures mental faculties, ensuring that the symphony of thoughts, memories, and reasoning remains vibrant and resilient throughout the years.

Exploring Cognitive Health: Strategies for Preservation

1. **Mental Stimulation:** Engage in activities that stimulate your mind, such as puzzles, games, or learning new skills. The brain thrives on novelty and challenges, and these activities contribute to the preservation of cognitive function.

2. **Healthy Nutrition**: Adopt a diet rich in brain-boosting nutrients, including omega-3 fatty acids, antioxidants, and vitamins. Foods like fatty fish, nuts, berries, and leafy greens nourish the brain and support its functions.

3. **Regular Exercise:** Physical activity is not only beneficial for the body but also for the mind. Exercise improves blood flow to the brain, promotes the growth of new neurons, and enhances cognitive function.

4. **Adequate Sleep**: Prioritize quality sleep as a crucial component of cognitive health. During sleep, the brain consolidates memories, clears toxins, and rejuvenates, contributing to optimal cognitive performance.

5. **Stress Management:** Chronic stress can adversely affect cognitive function. Adopt stress-reducing practices such as meditation, deep breathing, or mindfulness to cultivate a calm and resilient mind.

6. **Social Engagement**: Maintain meaningful social connections, as they play a significant role in preserving cognitive function. Regular social interactions contribute to emotional well-being and provide cognitive stimulation.

A Lifelong Commitment to Cognitive Resilience

Preserving your mind is not a one-time endeavor but a lifelong commitment to cognitive resilience. By incorporating these strategies into your daily life, you build a robust foundation that withstands the tests of time. As you age, your mind remains a beacon of brilliance, navigating the complexities of life with clarity, creativity, and wisdom.

So, fellow voyagers, let this chapter be your guide in the preservation of cognitive function—an exploration that celebrates the mind as the cornerstone of timeless brilliance. Onward to the nurturing of your mental sanctuary, where each thoughtful choice becomes a brushstroke in the masterpiece of aging with a mind that remains forever vibrant and brilliant!

Muscles

*Cultivating Muscular Vitality for Timeless Well-being***

In the symphony of aging gracefully, the chapter on preserving function unveils a key note—the significance of preserving muscle health. Let's unravel the importance of robust muscles for overall well-being and explore strategies that serve as a compass, guiding us to maintain muscle mass and strength throughout the journey of aging.

Preserving Your Muscles: The Pillars of Vitality

Muscles are not mere fibers that enable movement; they are the pillars of vitality, supporting overall health and functionality. Beyond the aesthetic aspects, robust muscles play a crucial role in daily activities, from carrying groceries to maintaining balance. Preserving muscle health becomes an investment in a life that not only spans years but is filled with vigor and mobility.

Why Muscle Preservation Matters: Beyond Aesthetics

Understanding the profound impact of muscle health on overall well-being is essential. Beyond aesthetics, preserved muscle mass contributes to metabolic health, helps maintain a healthy weight, and supports bone density. Strong muscles are the guardians of mobility, enabling an active and independent lifestyle as we navigate the passages of time.

Strategies for Muscular Vitality: Nurturing Strength Across Ages

Preserving muscle function is not an elusive quest but a journey that involves intentional choices and lifestyle habits. Here are strategies to nurture muscular vitality throughout the aging process:

1. **Resistance Training:** Engage in regular resistance or strength training exercises to challenge your muscles. This could involve lifting weights, using resistance bands, or performing bodyweight exercises. Resistance training stimulates muscle growth and strength.

2. **Balanced Nutrition:** Ensure your diet provides an adequate amount of protein, a key building block for muscles. A balanced intake of nutrients, including vitamins and minerals, supports overall muscle health.

3. **Hydration:** Stay well-hydrated, as water is essential for nutrient transport and overall cellular function, including muscle function.

4. **Adequate Rest:** Allow your muscles to recover by incorporating rest days into your exercise routine. Quality sleep is also crucial for muscle repair and growth.

5. **Flexibility Exercises:** Include flexibility exercises like yoga or stretching in your routine to maintain muscle flexibility and joint mobility.

6. **Regular Physical Activity:** Incorporate regular physical activity into your daily life. Even activities like walking, gardening, or dancing contribute to muscle health.

Cultivating Muscular Vitality for Old Age: A Lifelong Endeavor

Preserving your muscles is not a task reserved for a specific age; it's a lifelong endeavor. Whether you're in your twenties or well into your golden years, the choices you make today ripple through the tapestry of your future. By embracing strategies for muscular vitality, you lay the foundation for an old age where strength, mobility, and independence become cherished companions.

As we delve into the realm of preserving function, may the wisdom of nurturing muscle health guide us in aging with resilience and vitality. Onward to the exploration of strategies that become the guardians of muscular vitality, ensuring that the symphony of aging resonates with strength and well-being!

Sex Life

Nurturing Your Intimate Well-being

In the chapter dedicated to preserving function, the spotlight turns towards a topic that often carries a whisper of taboo—preserving your sex life as you age. This exploration extends beyond the physical realm, delving into the intricate interplay of factors that contribute to a healthy and satisfying sexual well-being. Let's unravel the secrets that nurture both the physical and emotional aspects of intimacy, paving the way for a fulfilling and vibrant sex life in the golden years.

Preserving Your Sex Life: A Journey Beyond Taboos

Embark on a journey that transcends societal taboos, where the preservation of your sex life becomes an essential facet of overall well-being. In the tapestry of aging, the intimate connection between partners is a thread that weaves joy, fulfillment, and a sense of vitality.

Physical Aspects: The Dance of Physiology

Explore the intricate dance of physiology, understanding how the physical aspects of aging can influence sexual well-being. From hormonal changes to the impact of chronic conditions, acknowledging and addressing these factors becomes a crucial step in preserving function. This journey involves open communication with healthcare professionals, paving the way for tailored solutions that align with individual needs.

Emotional Dimensions: Nurturing Intimacy

Delve into the emotional dimensions of preserving your sex life, recognizing the importance of intimacy in fostering emotional connection and well-being. Emotional intimacy becomes a cornerstone, enhancing the overall quality of relationships. Open communication, trust, and shared vulnerability contribute to a resilient foundation for maintaining a satisfying and vibrant sex life.

Communication is Key: A Bridge to Understanding

In the realm of preserving function, communication emerges as the key to understanding and navigating the changes that come with aging. Partners are encouraged to engage in open and honest conversations about desires, concerns, and expectations. This dialogue fosters a deeper connection, allowing both individuals to actively participate in the preservation of their sex life.

Professional Guidance: A Resource for Well-being

Seeking professional guidance, whether from healthcare professionals or sex therapists, becomes a valuable resource in the journey to preserve function. These experts can provide insights, address concerns, and offer tailored strategies to navigate the challenges that may arise. It's a proactive step towards ensuring that the intimate aspects of life remain fulfilling and satisfying.

As we navigate the terrain of preserving function, may this exploration into the intimate realm serve as a guide—a beacon illuminating the path to a fulfilling and vibrant sex life in the later years. By embracing the physical and emotional aspects, fostering open communication, and seeking professional support when needed, individuals can actively contribute to preserving their intimate well-being for a life that continues to bloom with joy and connection. Onward to the exploration of this essential aspect of aging, where the journey unfolds with grace and the embrace of lasting intimacy!

Skin

Nurturing Your Radiant Skin Through Time

In the chapter dedicated to preserving function, let's turn our attention to a canvas that often reflects the passage of time—our skin. Unveiling the secrets to maintaining healthy and radiant skin becomes an artful exploration, drawing from skincare practices, nutrition, and lifestyle habits that contribute to a timeless and youthful appearance.

Preserving Your Skin: A Symphony of Self-Care

Skincare Practices: Dive into the world of skincare practices as a form of self-care, where each ritual becomes a note in the symphony of preserving your skin. From gentle cleansing routines to the meticulous application of nourishing moisturizers and the protection offered by sunscreen, skincare practices contribute to maintaining the skin's health and resilience.

Nutrition: Explore the role of nutrition as a cornerstone in nurturing your skin from within. Antioxidant-rich foods, vitamins, and minerals play a crucial role in supporting collagen production, fighting oxidative stress, and promoting overall skin health. Embrace a diet that becomes a palette of nutrients, painting your skin with vitality and radiance.

Lifestyle Habits: Delve into lifestyle habits that become the brushstrokes in the canvas of preserving your skin. Prioritize hydration to keep your skin supple, embrace regular exercise to enhance blood flow and nourish your skin cells, and practice stress management to ward off the negative impacts of tension on your skin's appearance. Each habit becomes a pledge to nurture your skin through the ebb and flow of time.

A Ritual of Preservation: Aging Gracefully

Preserving your skin is not merely a task but a ritual—an intentional act of self-love and care. By incorporating skincare practices, embracing a skin-friendly diet, and cultivating lifestyle habits that prioritize your skin's well-being, you embark on a journey of aging gracefully.

As we unravel the secrets to preserving healthy and radiant skin, may this exploration inspire you to cultivate a skincare routine that transcends the surface and becomes a holistic approach to well-being. Each step becomes a gesture of preservation, ensuring that your skin, like a timeless masterpiece, reflects the beauty of aging gracefully. Onward to the exploration of preserving skin function—a celebration of self-care that transcends the hands of time!

Teeth

A Guide to Ageless Smiles

In the journey of preserving function, let's shine a spotlight on an often underestimated yet crucial aspect—oral health. This chapter unveils the secrets to maintaining strong and healthy teeth throughout the aging process. As we delve into preserving your teeth, effective strategies emerge as guardians, ensuring that your smile remains ageless.

Preserving Your Teeth: The Pillars of Oral Wellness

1. **Regular Dental Checkups:** Begin with the foundation—regular dental checkups. These appointments are not just for addressing existing issues but are preventive measures that catch potential problems in their infancy. Regular cleanings and examinations lay the groundwork for preserving your teeth.

2. **Effective Oral Hygiene Practices:** Embrace effective oral hygiene practices as daily rituals. Brushing your teeth twice a day with fluoride toothpaste and using dental floss to clean between teeth are simple yet powerful habits. These practices remove plaque, prevent cavities, and contribute to the overall health of your gums.

3. Balanced Diet for Dental Health: Nourish your teeth from within by adopting a balanced diet. Incorporate foods rich in calcium, such as dairy products and leafy greens, for strong teeth and bones. Limit sugary snacks and beverages, as they can contribute to tooth decay.

4. Hydration and Saliva Production: Stay hydrated for the sake of your oral health. Adequate water intake promotes saliva production, which plays a crucial role in neutralizing acids, cleansing the mouth, and remineralizing teeth. A well-hydrated mouth is a resilient fortress against decay.

5. Avoidance of Harmful Habits: Bid farewell to harmful habits that can compromise your teeth. Smoking and excessive alcohol consumption not only harm your overall health but can also have detrimental effects on your oral well-being. Kick these habits for a brighter and healthier smile.

6. Protection Against Grinding: If you grind your teeth, consider protective measures such as a mouthguard. Grinding, especially during sleep, can wear down enamel and lead to various dental issues. Preserving function involves addressing potential threats, and a mouthguard can be a safeguard against grinding-related damage.

7. **Prompt Addressing of Dental Issues:** Don't ignore dental issues; address them promptly. Whether it's a toothache, sensitivity, or any other concern, swift action can prevent further damage. Regular

communication with your dentist ensures that issues are caught early, preserving the function and aesthetics of your teeth.

As we navigate the path of preserving function, let oral health take center stage. By incorporating these strategies into your daily routine, you not only preserve your teeth but also contribute to your overall well-being. A bright, healthy smile is not just a reflection of good oral health but a timeless asset that accompanies you on the journey of graceful aging. Onward to the exploration of preserving your teeth— a key to an ageless and vibrant smile!

Vision

Nurturing the Windows to the Soul

In the symphony of aging gracefully, the chapter on preserving function emerges as a testament to the care we can bestow upon the intricate components of our bodies. Let's delve into the delicate realm of eye health, unveiling the intricacies of preserving and supporting optimal vision as we gracefully navigate the golden years.

Preserving Your Vision: A Journey into Eye Health

Embark on a journey into the world of eye health—a precious facet of preserving function as we age. Our eyes, the windows to the soul, deserve the utmost care and attention. The complexities of vision involve not only the eyes themselves but also the intricate connections to the brain that shape our perception of the world.

Nurturing Optimal Vision: A Lifelong Endeavor

Preserving and supporting optimal vision is not a task reserved for a specific age; it's a lifelong endeavor. The choices we make today contribute to the clarity of our vision tomorrow. From nutrition to protective measures, understanding the factors that influence eye health becomes a compass guiding us on the path to preserving function.

Understanding the Intricacies: Aging and Vision

As we gracefully age, the intricacies of vision evolve. Conditions such as presbyopia, macular degeneration, and cataracts may become more prevalent. Yet, armed with knowledge and proactive measures, we can mitigate the impact of these changes and foster a vision that remains sharp and clear.

Nutrition for Eye Health: Feeding the Windows to the Soul

Explore the role of nutrition in nurturing eye health. Foods rich in antioxidants, vitamins, and minerals contribute to the well-being of our eyes. From leafy greens to vibrant fruits, the palette of nutrients becomes a canvas upon which we paint the hues of optimal vision.

Protective Measures: Safeguarding the Gift of Sight

In the realm of preserving vision, protective measures become our guardians. Whether it's wearing sunglasses to shield against harmful UV rays or practicing the 20-20-20 rule to alleviate eye strain in the digital age, these measures add layers of protection to the windows of our soul.

Regular Eye Checkups: A Ritual of Care

As a ritual of care, regular eye checkups become a cornerstone of preserving function. These checkups not only detect potential issues early but also provide an opportunity to discuss any changes in vision and receive guidance on maintaining optimal eye health.

In the tapestry of aging, the chapter on preserving function—specifically, preserving your vision—becomes a poignant ode to the gift of sight. With knowledge as our guide and proactive measures as our tools, we navigate the journey with eyes that not only see the world but also witness the beauty of aging with clarity and grace. Onward to the exploration of eye health, where each choice becomes a step toward preserving the windows to the soul!

Dignity

Nurturing Dignity in the Tapestry of Aging

As we conclude the exploration of preserving function in the journey of aging, a poignant chapter unfolds—*Preserving Your Dignity*. Here, we delve into the intrinsic importance of maintaining dignity as a central aspect of aging well. In the intricate tapestry of life, emotional and psychological well-being takes center stage, serving as the essence of preserving one's sense of self and worth.

Nurturing Emotional Resilience: A Pillar of Dignity

Emotional resilience becomes a pillar supporting the preservation of dignity. As we age, facing the inevitable changes and challenges, the ability to adapt emotionally becomes paramount. This resilience is not about suppressing emotions but navigating them with grace, acknowledging the evolving nature of life while preserving the core of one's emotional well-being.

Cultivating Psychological Well-being: The Inner Garden of Dignity

The garden of psychological well-being flourishes when tended with care. It involves embracing self-awareness, fostering a positive mindset, and seeking support when needed. As we age, the inner landscape becomes a sanctuary where the seeds of self-worth are sown, and the blooms of a resilient psyche flourish. Cultivating this garden is an intentional act, ensuring that the roots of one's dignity run deep.

Empowering Independence: A Gateway to Dignity

Preserving dignity in old age is intertwined with maintaining a sense of independence. Empowering oneself in daily tasks, seeking assistance when required, and making choices that align with personal values contribute to a continued sense of autonomy. Independence becomes a gateway to dignity, allowing individuals to shape their own narratives even as the chapters of life unfold.

Building Meaningful Connections: The Tapestry of Dignity Woven with Others

Dignity is not a solitary endeavor but a collaborative masterpiece woven through meaningful connections with others. Building and maintaining relationships, be it with family, friends, or community, creates a network of support. These connections become threads in the tapestry of dignity, providing strength and companionship throughout the aging journey.

Acknowledging Life Transitions: A Compassionate Approach to Dignity

As we age, life transitions become inevitable. Whether it's retirement, changes in health, or shifts in roles, acknowledging these transitions with a compassionate lens fosters dignity. Embracing the ebb and flow of life's phases, while maintaining a sense of purpose, contributes to a dignified existence.

In the symphony of preserving function, the melody of dignity resonates as a central note. It's an ongoing composition, requiring intentional choices and nurturing. As we wrap up this chapter, let's celebrate the significance of preserving one's dignity—an artful endeavor that enhances the quality of life and ensures that the journey of aging is adorned with grace, self-worth, and a profound sense of dignity. Onward to the exploration of aging well, where each step is an affirmation of preserving function with dignity as our guiding light!

Chapter 3 provides a holistic approach to preserving various bodily functions, offering practical advice for readers to maintain their overall well-being. If you have any specific preferences or if you'd like further adjustments, feel free to let me know!

IV. Dr. Greger's Anti-Aging Essentials

Symphony for Graceful Aging

As we step into the realm of ageless vitality, a compelling chapter unfolds—*Dr. Greger's Anti-Aging Essentials*. At its heart lies the promise of a healthy and vibrant life, encapsulated in the Anti-Aging Eight—a collection of essential elements meticulously curated by Dr. Greger. Let the curtain rise as we embark on a journey to explore these scientifically-backed strategies, each note in this symphony resonating as a guide for aging gracefully.

Setting the Stage: The Overture of Essential Elements

In this symphony of health and longevity, the overture introduces Dr. Greger's Anti-Aging Eight—an ensemble of strategies designed to harmonize with the natural rhythms of aging. This collection serves not only as a guide but as a testament to the power of science-backed choices in shaping a graceful and vibrant journey through the years.

The Anti-Aging Eight Unveiled: A Prelude to Vitality

Dr. Greger's Anti-Aging Eight unfolds like a well-composed prelude, each element playing a distinctive role in the pursuit of ageless well-being:

1. **Nuts:** A symphony of essential nutrients and heart-healthy fats, nuts become the foundational note for vitality

2. **Greens:** The verdant greens take center stage, offering a chorus of antioxidants, vitamins, and minerals, supporting the body's resilience.

3. **Berries:** Like a melodic refrain, berries add a burst of flavor and a plethora of phytonutrients, contributing to cellular health and vibrancy.

4. **Xenohormesis and Microrna Manipulation:** A nuanced movement in the symphony, exploring the interplay of environmental stressors and microRNA manipulation—a key to unlocking the secrets of longevity.

5. **Prebiotics and Postbiotics:** The rhythm of gut health reverberates, with prebiotics and postbiotics orchestrating a harmonious dance in support of overall well-being.

6. **Caloric Restriction:** A gentle modulation in the tempo, caloric restriction emerges as a strategic choice, influencing the aging process at a cellular level.

7. **Protein Restriction:** A deliberate modulation of protein intake becomes a refined note, contributing to the balance in Dr. Greger's symphony for graceful aging.

8. **NAD+:** The grand crescendo—the essential role of NAD+ in cellular energy metabolism, unveiling a key element in the pursuit of vitality.

A Melody for the Ages: Exploring the Anti-Aging Eight

As we embark on this exploration, each element in Dr. Greger's Anti-Aging Eight becomes a note in a melody for the ages. Together, they compose a symphony that resonates with the principles of science, the wisdom of nature, and the artistry of aging gracefully.

May this chapter be a beacon of knowledge, guiding us toward a life that embraces the Anti-Aging Eight—a life that ages not just with the passage of time but with the grace of well-informed choices. Onward to the exploration of Dr. Greger's Anti-Aging Essentials, where each note is an invitation to dance through the years with vitality, health, and the timeless beauty of graceful aging!